NATURAL WELLNESS TECHNIQUES FOR WOMEN

Strategies To Help Women Stay Healthy And Balanced

By
Eugene Williams

Table of contents

Introduction

Welcome to "Natural Wellness techniques for Women," a thorough manual whose goal is to provide women with the information and resources they need to put their health and well-being first using all-natural methods. The significance of natural well-being for women in the fast-paced world of today cannot be emphasized. Women take on a variety of duties, often juggling families, professions, and countless other obligations, making their health a top priority.

1. Natural Wellness is Important for Women:

Women have distinct physiological changes in their bodies throughout their lives, from adolescence through menopause and beyond. Numerous physical and mental health issues may result from these changes. Understanding these special features and implementing natural wellness practices that cater to our bodies' requirements are the keys to attaining maximum well-being.

2. The Ebook's Purpose and Objectives:

This book's main goal is to become your dependable travel partner for discovering natural healing. Our mission is to provide you with insightful knowledge, factual data, and useful guidance so you can naturally take control of your health. We provide information on everything from diet to exercise to stress reduction to hormonal balance to skincare to aging gracefully.

3. A Quick Summary of What Readers Can Anticipate

The complexity of women's health will be covered in detail in the subsequent chapters, which will cover everything from identifying the particular health issues that women face to developing individualized wellness programs. You may anticipate learning:

- **Chapter 1:** A look at the special characteristics of women's health and how natural wellness may help with these issues.

- **Chapter 2:** Nutritional insights, including information on the value of a balanced diet, essential nutrients for women's health, and useful recipes.

- **Chapter 3:** Advice on fitness and exercise adapted to various life phases.

- **Chapter 4:** Techniques for reducing stress and fostering mental health.

- **Chapter 5:** In-depth discussion of menstrual health and hormone balance.

- **Chapter 6:** Natural skin care advice for preserving healthy, radiant skin.

-**Chapter 7:** offers advice on aging gracefully and keeping your energy.

- **Chapter 8:** provides an overview of herbal treatments and dietary supplements for women's health.

- **Chapter 9:** How to build a unique natural health strategy.

Resources and further reading for ongoing education and assistance are covered in Chapter 10.

- **Chapter 11:** A summary of the most important ideas and a call to action on your road to well-being.

By the time you finish reading this booklet, you will have the information and resources necessary to start a natural health path that is specifically designed for the requirements of women. We're here to help you every step of the way as you make natural health and well-being your top priorities. Together, let's start this empowering adventure.

Chapter 1

Understanding Women's Health

We will set out on a journey to enhance our awareness of women's health in this chapter, reviewing the distinctive characteristics that characterize it, the typical health issues that women experience, and how natural wellness practices may successfully treat these issues.

1. Distinctive Elements of Women's Health

The unique characteristics of women's health are influenced by the intricate interaction of biology, genetics, and hormonal changes. It's critical to recognize the following to properly understand their distinctive characteristics:

- **Hormonal variations include:** Throughout their lives, women undergo a variety of hormonal changes, from puberty and menstruation through pregnancy, postpartum, and menopause. These changes have an impact on general health as well as reproductive health.

- **Healthy Reproduction:** Reproductive health is essential since only women possess reproductive organs including the uterus and ovaries. It is essential to comprehend the menstrual cycle, fertility, and available forms of contraception.

• Bone health Due to hormonal fluctuations, women are more vulnerable to diseases like osteoporosis, which highlights the need for calcium consumption and weight-bearing workouts.

• Breast Health For women, breast cancer is a serious problem. Mammograms and regular breast self-examinations are essential for early detection.

2. Typical Health Issues for Women:

A variety of health issues that women face might influence their quality of life. Among the most common problems are:

Menstrual disorders are as follows: Conditions including painful menstruation, heavy periods, and erratic cycles may interfere with everyday living.

• **Polycystic Ovary Syndrome (PCOS)**

A hormonal disease that affects many women and may impact fertility.

   Menopause symptoms include: Women may have hot flashes, mood fluctuations, and changes in bone density as menopause approaches.

   - Mental Health Women are more prone to mental illnesses including sadness and anxiety, which are often related to hormonal changes and phases of life.

   -Heart and Vascular Health: Women are more likely to die from heart disease than males, thus it is important to practice heart-healthy practices.

3. The Contribution of Natural Wellness to Solving These Problems

Natural wellness strategies are ideally adapted to efficiently address the particular elements of women's health and treat common health issues. ***This is how:***

- Natural Methods for Hormone Balancing

Natural methods including stress management, a healthy diet, regular exercise, and herbal therapies may help control hormonal swings and lessen menstrual, PCOS, and menopausal symptoms.

- Nutritional Support for Women's Health

While phytoestrogens and antioxidants included in plant-based foods help to maintain hormonal balance, a diet high in these nutrients may benefit bone health.

- Mind-Body Techniques: Deep breathing exercises, yoga, and mindfulness meditation are among the methods that may help you manage stress, enhance your mental health, and lower your risk of cardiovascular disease.

   - **Holistic health:** Women may be empowered to take control of their health and make wise choices by adopting a holistic approach to health that considers their physical, mental, and emotional well-being.

The first step in implementing natural wellness practices that might result in a happier, more balanced existence is understanding the particular elements of women's health and identifying prevalent difficulties. The next chapters will go further into certain facets of women's wellbeing and provide you with helpful advice and doable actions to improve your path to natural wellness.

Chapter 2

Diet and Nutrition

We will examine the crucial part that food and nutrition play in women's health in this chapter. We'll talk about the value of eating a balanced diet, highlight important nutrients for women's health, and provide you with useful meal plans and recipes to help you on your path to natural well-being.

1. The significance of a balanced diet:

For women, eating a balanced diet consistently is essential to optimal health. *Here is why it's important:*

- **General Health:** Your body receives the vital vitamins, minerals, and nutrients it needs from a balanced diet to operate at its best. It promotes high energy levels, sharp cognitive ability, and a robust immune system.

- **Hormonal Harmony:** A balanced diet that contains certain nutrients may help control hormonal changes and lessen menstrual and menopausal symptoms.

- **Bone health** A healthy diet rich in calcium and vitamin D promotes strong bones and lowers the risk of osteoporosis.

- **Heart Condition:** A diet rich in fiber and low in saturated fats may help women's cardiovascular health, a major issue.

2. Important Foods for Women's Health

Throughout their lives, women have varying nutritional demands. The following essential nutrients are particularly important for women's health:

  - **Calcium:** Calcium-rich meals, such as dairy products, leafy greens, and fortified plant-based substitutes, are crucial for bone health.

  - **Iron:** Women require iron to avoid anemia, particularly throughout the reproductive years. Lean meats, beans, and fortified cereals are among the sources.

  - **Folate:** Leafy greens, beans, and fortified cereals all contain folate, which is essential during pregnancy to avoid birth abnormalities

Omega-3 Fatty Acids: These fats may be derived from fatty fish, flaxseeds, and walnuts and help both heart health and cognitive function.

   -- Vitamin D: which is required for the absorption of calcium, may be received from food sources including fortified dairy or plant-based milk as well as sunshine.

3. Natural Wellness Recipes and Meal Plans:

Here, we provide you with useful tools to develop a healthy diet that is wholesome and well-balanced:

   - Recipe suggestions: Find tasty, simple-to-make meals that include nutrient-dense foods. We've chosen a variety of meals that suit a variety of tastes and dietary needs, from robust salads to healthful soups and smoothie bowls.

- Examples of Meal Plans Pregnancy, menopause, and post-menopause are just a few of the life periods for which we've produced example meal plans. You may more easily achieve your nutritional requirements thanks to these programs' recommendations for serving sizes and nutrient consumption.

  - Plant-Based Alternatives: To help you maintain your health and well-being while consuming a plant-based diet, we've also included plant-based meal suggestions that are packed with the nutrients that women need.

  - Lists of Things to Buy: We've created shopping lists that are specific to meal plans to make grocery shopping simple and help you on your path to a healthy diet.

We provide you with the tools you need to make educated food decisions that support your natural wellness objectives by emphasizing the significance of a balanced diet, highlighting important nutrients for women's health, and offering useful resources like recipes, meal plans, and shopping lists. A healthy body is better able to handle life's obstacles, and it's an essential step on the road to happiness and health.

Chapter 3

Exercise and Fitness

This chapter will examine the role that fitness and exercise play in a woman's quest for natural well-being. We'll explore the advantages of regular exercise, thc bcst exercises for various life phases, and how to design a tailored fitness program that meets your specific requirements and objectives.

The advantages of regular exercise for women include:

Regular physical exercise has a host of advantages, many of which are beneficial to women's health:

Heart and Vascular Health: By lowering the risk of heart disease, high blood pressure, and stroke, exercise improves heart health.

- **Weight Control:** A healthy weight is essential for general well-being and the avoidance of chronic diseases, and regular exercise helps maintain a healthy weight.

- **Mental and Mood Health:** Exercise improves mental health by releasing endorphins, which lessen stress, anxiety, and depressive symptoms.

Weight-bearing activities like walking and resistance training promote bone density and lower the risk of osteoporosis.

 - **Hormonal Harmony:** Exercise may help control hormonal swings and alleviate menstrual and menopausal symptoms.

 - **Better Sleep:** Regular exercise may improve sleep length and quality, which benefits overall vitality.

Exercises to Perform at Different Life Stages:

The best kind of exercise differs depending on your stage of life, thus it's important to choose exercises that fit your requirements and talents precisely:

Young Adulthood: Building a solid foundation for fitness and general health may be accomplished via exercises like jogging, cycling, and weight training.

- **Miscarriage:** Swimming, low-impact aerobics, and prenatal yoga may all help you stay healthy throughout pregnancy while lowering your risk.

After giving birth: Walking, pelvic floor exercises, and other gentle workouts help with recuperation and a gradual return to fitness.

- **Menopause**: Taijiquan, yoga, and weight-bearing activities may support bone density and regulate hormonal fluctuations.

- The "Golden Years" Swimming, water aerobics, and tai chi are all low-impact exercises that are great for preserving mobility.

3. Designing a Customized Fitness Program:

For long-term success, it's crucial to create a fitness plan that is appropriate to your requirements and objectives. Here is a step-by-step instruction sheet to get you going:

- **Determine Your Objectives:** Decide what you want to accomplish with exercise, such as bettering your cardiovascular health, losing weight, reducing stress, or gaining more strength and flexibility.

- **Consider Your Preferences:** Pick activities you find enjoyable to boost the probability that you will continue your exercise regimen.

-**Begin Sluggishly:** Start with low-intensity exercises and gradually increase the time and intensity, especially if you're new to exercising or coming back after a hiatus.

- **Incorporate Variety:** Include a variety of exercises to improve balance, flexibility, strength, and endurance.

- **Set Realistic Goals:** To remain motivated, set realistic benchmarks and monitor your progress.

- **Prioritize Safety:** Before beginning a new fitness regimen, particularly if you have underlying medical concerns, speak with a healthcare professional.

- **Listen to Your Body:** Pay attention to how your body reacts to exercise and modify your program as necessary to avoid injury or overexertion.

- **Maintain Consistency:** To experience the long-term advantages of exercise, consistency is essential. Aim for consistent, sustained exercise that fits into your daily routine.

You are moving much closer to natural well-being by realizing the advantages of regular exercise, choosing activities that are appropriate for your stage of life, and developing a customized fitness regimen. Exercise is important for overall well-being, which enables you to live a full and active life. It isn't simply for physical health.

Chapter 4

Mental Health and Stress Management

The vital subject of stress management and mental health will be covered in this chapter, with an emphasis on understanding stress and how it affects women's health, going through natural stress-reduction techniques, and advocating for general mental wellness.

1. Recognizing Stress and How It Affects Women's Health

Modern life is filled with stress, which may have a negative influence on the health of women. The first step to successfully managing stress is to comprehend the relationship between it and well-being:

 - *Physical effects include:* Physical symptoms including headaches, digestive issues, and a weaker immune system may result from prolonged stress. Long-term, it may aggravate issues including heart disease and high blood pressure.

 - *Emotional Effects* Anxiety, irritation, and depressive moods are often brought on by stress. Due to hormonal changes, women may be more susceptible to these emotional reactions.

- **Hormonal Alterations:** Long-term stress may throw off the body's hormonal balance, which might lead to irregular menstruation, worsen menopausal symptoms, and affect fertility.

Sleep disturbances include: Sleep problems brought on by stress may hurt mood, cognition, and general health.

2. Natural Techniques for Reducing Stress

Adopting healthy routines and techniques that benefit your body and mind is a natural way to combat stress. Here are a few sensible ideas:

- **Meditation and Mindfulness:** You may improve your capacity for stress management, remain present, and minimize anxiety with the aid of these techniques.

  - **Yoga:** Yoga blends physical postures with breathing techniques, meditation, and stress reduction.

  - **Physical Exercise:** Exercise regularly to relieve stress by releasing endorphins, your body's natural mood enhancers.

  - Deep breathing exercises Deep, diaphragmatic breathing exercises help relax the nervous system and lessen stress.

  -- Aromatherapy Lavender and chamomile are two examples of essential oils that have soothing effects and may be used in aromatherapy to promote relaxation.

  Teas made from herbs and Herbs like chamomile, valerian root, and passionflower may be found in teas that are relaxing.

3. Promoting Mental Health:

For general health and stress resistance, taking care of your mental health is crucial:

•Prioritize self-care practices like reading, taking baths, and spending time in nature that make you feel happy and relaxed.

• Maintaining close relationships with friends and family is important because they provide you with emotional support and a feeling of community.

Seeking Expert Assistance: Do not be reluctant to seek help from a therapist, counselor, or support group if stress becomes unbearable or negatively impacts your mental health.

Healthy Lifestyle Decisions: To promote mental health, a balanced diet, frequent exercise, and enough sleep are all essential.

 - **Time Management:** Manage your time well to relieve stress caused by demanding schedules and obligations.

You may improve your resilience, emotional balance, and general quality of life by being aware of how stress affects women's health, adopting natural stress-reduction techniques into your routine, and actively supporting mental wellness. To achieve holistic health as a woman, stress management is essential. It is also a cornerstone of natural well-being.

Chapter 5

Menstrual Health and Hormone Balance

We will dig into the complex realm of hormone balance and menstrual health in this chapter. Your natural wellness path must include learning about the hormonal shifts that occur in women's bodies, investigating all-natural methods of controlling hormonal imbalances, and learning techniques for a regular menstrual cycle.

1. Changes in Women's Bodies Caused by Hormones

From adolescence through menopause, women's bodies experience considerable hormonal changes. Various biological systems, including reproduction, are regulated by these changes:

- **Menstruation Cycle:** Ovulation and menstruation are caused by changes in estrogen and progesterone levels, which regulate the menstrual cycle.

- **Prudence:** Hormonal changes that result in breast growth, the start of menstruation, and the emergence of secondary sexual traits signal the beginning of puberty.

- **Miscarriage:** A successful pregnancy, including the growth of the placenta and preservation of the uterine lining, depends on hormonal changes.

   menopause Declining levels of estrogen and progesterone, which cause menstruation to stop and other symptoms, mark the onset of menopause.

Natural Methods for Treating Hormonal Imbalances:

The therapy of disorders like polycystic ovarian syndrome (PCOS) or irregular menstrual periods depends on maintaining hormonal balance. *Here are some organic tactics to take into account:*

• **Balanced diet** A diet high in whole foods, such as fruits, vegetables, whole grains, and lean meats, may maintain hormone balance and help manage insulin levels.

• **Stress management** Hormonal equilibrium may be disturbed by high amounts of stress. Include methods for reducing stress in your routine, such as yoga, meditation, and deep breathing exercises.

- **Herbal Treatments:** Traditional uses of several herbs, including black cohosh and chasteberry (Vitex agnus-castus), enhance hormonal balance. Before utilizing herbal medicines, get medical advice.

Regular Exercise: Exercise may promote healthy hormone function and aid in managing insulin.

•**Getting enough sleep** Prioritize getting good sleep since it may alter how your hormones are produced and regulated.

3. Methods for Maintaining a Healthy Menstrual Cycle:

A regular menstrual cycle is a sign of hormonal balance and reproductive health. *The following are methods to promote menstrual health:*

Nutritionally Rich Diet: A diet high in key nutrients may lower the risk of anemia and maintain a regular menstrual cycle, notably iron and B vitamins.

- Hydroponics: Bloating and pain during menstruation may be reduced by drinking plenty of water.

- Products for Menstrual Care: Consider natural and environmentally friendly period care choices like menstrual cups or reusable cloth pads.

- Pain Management: Herbal supplements (such as turmeric) and heat treatment are examples of natural medicines that may aid with menstrual pain relief.

• **Monitoring Your Cycle:** You may better understand your body's natural pattern by keeping a monthly cycle journal, which will make it simpler to spot any changes or anomalies that may need your attention.

You may take charge of your reproductive health and general well-being as a woman by being aware of hormonal shifts, using natural methods to treat hormonal imbalances, and putting healthy menstrual cycle tactics into practice. This information gives you the power to adopt natural health activities that are in line with your hormonal requirements and to make educated decisions.

Chapter 6

Skin and Beauty

This chapter will look at natural wellness tactics that women may use to preserve beautiful, healthy skin and accentuate their inherent attractiveness. We'll talk about chemical-free ways to improve your appearance, address healthy skincare regimens, and provide advice for beautiful, healthy skin.

1. Women's Natural Skincare Routines

A natural skincare regimen may assist you in achieving and maintaining a beautiful complexion since your skin is a reflection of your general health. *How to begin going is as follows:*

  - **Cleansing:** To clean your skin without robbing it of its natural oils, use mild, natural cleansers.

  -- **Exfoliation** Use natural exfoliants to remove dead skin cells and reveal a glowing, fresh complexion, such as sugar, oats, or clay masks.

  - **Hydration:** Pick natural moisturizers with nourishing components like aloe vera, jojoba oil, or shea butter for your skin.

  - **Sun Protection:** Use mineral-based sunscreens and wear protective gear to shield your skin from UV rays.

  - **Natural Substances:** Look for skincare products that include components like chamomile, rosehip oil, or tea tree oil, which are recognized for their calming effects on the skin.

2. Advice for Having Healthy and Gleaming Skin:

Beyond using skincare products, you may achieve and keep beautiful, healthy skin. *Here are some more ideas to think about:*

  - **Hydration:** To keep your skin moisturized from the inside out and promote a glowing complexion, drink lots of water.

- **Balanced Diet:** Fruits and vegetables, which are nutrient-rich foods, include important vitamins and antioxidants that promote the health of the skin.

Enough Sleep: Make sure you obtain enough amount of restful sleep, since this is essential for skin renewal and restoration.

- **Stress management** Manage your tension with breathing exercises, yoga, or meditation to stop skin problems from becoming worse from stress.

Regular Exercise: Exercise encourages wholesome circulation, which may make your skin shine.

3. Enhancing Natural Beauty Without Negative Chemicals:

No dangerous substances or intrusive procedures are necessary to enhance your natural attractiveness. How to appreciate your individual beauty while keeping it natural is provided here:

- **Little to No Makeup:** Choose cosmetics that don't include harsh chemicals, parabens, or artificial perfumes. Instead of hiding natural traits, emphasize them.

- **Healthy Hair Maintenance:** Pick natural hair products that nourish your hair without adding any hazardous ingredients. Regular cuts and delicate style techniques may also support the preservation of healthy hair.

- **Body self-assurance:** Recognize that beauty comes in many forms and sizes and accept your body as it is. Put your attention on feeling secure and at ease in your own flesh.

- A positive self-perception: Practice self-compassion and self-acceptance to develop a good self-image. Be in the company of individuals who enhance and support your sense of self.

You may take care of your skin and general well-being by implementing natural skincare regimens, following advice for healthy, bright skin, and enhancing your natural beauty without the use of damaging chemicals. Keep in mind that genuine beauty comes from inside and that your path toward natural healing offers you the chance to improve both your inner and exterior attractiveness as a woman.

Chapter 7

Growing Old With Grace

We'll talk about how to age gracefully as a woman in this chapter. We'll talk about how important it is to accept aging, provide natural anti-aging cures, and offer advice on how to stay healthy as you go through different phases of life.

1. Acknowledging the Aging Process

Being happy about aging is crucial since aging is a normal and unavoidable aspect of life:

  - **Self-Acceptance:** Accept your age-related changes, such as wrinkles, gray hair, and changing body types. These are indications of a full existence.

  Knowledge and Experience: Age brings with it experience and wisdom. Celebrate your successes and the wisdom you've acquired over the years.

  •Prioritize self-care activities that take into account your changing requirements, with a particular emphasis on your physical and emotional well-being.

2. Natural remedies and anti-aging advice

While you cannot turn back the hands of time, you may develop behaviors that decrease the negative consequences of aging and support healthy aging.

Nutritionally Rich Diet: To maintain your skin, bones, and general health, keep placing a high priority on eating a balanced diet that is rich in antioxidants, vitamins, and minerals.

- Hydration: Keep your body well hydrated to preserve organ and skin flexibility.

- Practice: You may preserve bone density, muscular tone, and general vigor by engaging in regular physical exercise.

- Sun Protection: To prevent early aging and lower your risk of skin cancer, keep protecting your skin from the sun with clothes and sunscreen.

- Stress Reduction: Stress management is even more essential for general health as you become older. Investigate methods of relaxation such as mindfulness, meditation, or mild yoga.

 - **Quality Rest:** Give peaceful sleep a priority to help both physical and mental renewal.

 - **Natural skincare:** Take into account employing hydrating, collagen-producing, and skin-healthy natural skincare products.

 - **Supplements:** Speak to a healthcare professional about supplements like collagen or vitamins B12 and D that may help with aging.

3. Keeping Women's Vitality as They Age:

The secret to aging well is to maintain your vitality. *Here are some tips to maintain and improve your vitality:*

- **Mental Fitness:** Take part in mental-strengthening activities like crossword puzzles, reading, or picking up new skills.

- **Social Relationships:** To prevent isolation and loneliness, which may harm one's mental and emotional health, stay in touch with friends and family.

- **Physical Exercise:** Regular exercise improves mood and general vigor while also maintaining physical health.

- **Purpose:** Look for activities and projects that give your life significance, whether via charitable work, a hobby, or artistic interests.

Regular health examinations: To identify and manage health concerns early, keep setting up routine checkups and screenings with healthcare professionals.

Positive Outlook: Develop a positive outlook on aging by seeing it as a chance for development and new experiences.

The process of graceful aging may be powerful and gratifying. You may keep a healthy, meaningful life at any point by accepting aging, using natural anti-aging therapies, and concentrating on sustaining energy. Keep in mind that age is only a number and that the energy and pleasure you bring to each day is the ultimate test of your well-being.

Chapter 8

Supplements and Herbal Treatments

The world of herbal remedies and supplements will be explored in this chapter, along with an introduction to herbal medicine, a discussion of popular herbs and supplements for women's health, and an emphasis on the necessity of following safety precautions and usage instructions when incorporating them into your natural wellness routine.

1. An Overview of Herbal Medicine

Herbal medicine is a tried-and-true method for using plants' inherent ability to cure to promote health and well-being. By treating the underlying causes of health problems, it provides a comprehensive approach to well-being. ***What you need to know is as follows:***

- Conventional Wisdom Across nations, herbal treatments have been utilized for ages, using the knowledge of earlier times.

- **Holistic Approach:** When treating health issues, herbal medicine takes the complete person—physical, emotional, and spiritual—into account.

- **Additional Care:** Supplementing traditional medical procedures with herbal therapies may help boost women's health.

2. Typical Supplements and Herbs for Women's Health

The potential advantages of several herbs and supplements in treating different women's health issues have come to light. *Here are a few that are often used:*

•Chantecaille (Vitex agnus-castus) Chasteberry, which can balance hormones, is used to treat monthly irregularities, PMS, and menopausal symptoms.

•Black cohosh Hot flashes and mood swings associated with menopause are often treated with this medication.

-Evening Primrose Oil: This supplement, which is high in gamma-linolenic acid (GLA), may improve skin health and help control hormonal imbalances.

- Phytoestrogens found in red clover may help with menopausal symptoms.

- **Dong Quai:** used in traditional Chinese medicine to treat menstruation irregularities and symptoms of menopause.

- **Saw palmetto:** Occasionally advised for promoting female reproductive and urinary health.

- **St. John's Wort:** Known for having the ability to lessen mild to moderate depressive and anxiety symptoms.

- **Turmeric:** It has anti-inflammatory properties and may benefit joint health as well as general wellness.

- **Iron:** Vital for women with anemia who are low in iron, particularly during menstruation or pregnancy.

 - **Vitamin D and calcium** are crucial for maintaining bone health, particularly as women age.

 -**Folate:** Essential for preventing birth abnormalities during pregnancy.

Guidelines for Safety and Appropriate Use:

While using herbal medicines and supplements carefully and sensibly might have potential benefits:

Consult a healthcare professional. Consult a healthcare professional before beginning any new herbal cure or supplement, particularly if you have underlying medical issues, are pregnant, or are breastfeeding.

Dosage and quality: To guarantee safety and efficacy, stick to suggested doses and choose reputed, high-quality products.

- **Possible interactions:** Be mindful of any possible drug interactions you may be taking. With your healthcare practitioner, go through them.

- **Keep an eye out for allergies:** Keep an eye out for any allergic reactions or negative side effects, and stop using the product if they do.

- **Continuity:** Be consistent with use to gauge the efficacy of any herbal treatments or supplements you decide to add to your health regimen.

- **Educate Yourself:** Take the time to educate yourself on the herbs and supplements you want to take, including any possible advantages and disadvantages.

Herbal cures and supplements may be helpful tools in your quest for natural well-being, but you should take them with caution and under a doctor's supervision. They may effectively assist women's health by treating a variety of issues and fostering general well-being when addressed carefully.

Chapter 10

Building a Natural Wellness Plan

We'll walk you through the process of developing a natural health plan that is unique to you as a woman and is suited to your requirements and objectives in this chapter. On your path to health, we'll go through how to create objectives that matter, monitor your progress wisely, and maintain accountability.

1. Developing a Customized Wellness Plan:

The road map for your natural health journey is a well-structured wellness plan. This is how you make one:

- **Evaluation:** Start by evaluating your present state of health and well-being. Think about your life's physical, mental, and emotional aspects. Determine any areas that want development or particular objectives you'd like to accomplish.

- **Prioritize Your Goals:** Choose your main wellness concerns. These could include stress reduction, maintaining a healthy weight, developing physical fitness, or promoting mental well-being.

- **Natural Techniques:** Investigate the natural health techniques covered in earlier chapters that fit your objectives. Consider adding mindfulness or yoga to your regimen, for example, if managing your stress is your top concern.

- **Customization:** Adjust your strategy to suit your tastes and way of life. Because consistency is essential for success, make sure it's attainable and long-lasting.

2. Setting Objectives and Monitoring Progress:

Success requires establishing definite, attainable objectives and monitoring your progress. Here's an efficient way to go about it:

- **Clear and Measurable Objectives:** Clear up your objectives. Set a specific objective, such as "practice mindfulness meditation for 15 minutes every day," as opposed to a general one like "reduce stress."

- **Timeline:** Decide on a reasonable timetable for completing each objective.

Take into account both immediate and long-term goals.

- **Tracking Instruments:** To keep track of your progress, use tools like notebooks, apps, or calendars. Keep a journal of your activities, any alterations in your routines, and any changes in your mood.

- **Celebrate Milestones:** Take time to recognize and appreciate your progress. Small successes might give you the drive to go on.

- **Adjust as necessary:** Be willing to change your strategy as needed. Don't give up if you run into problems or have to change course because of the situation. Adapt your objectives and tactics as necessary.

3. Maintaining Motivation and Accountability

Although maintaining accountability and motivation might be difficult, it is crucial for long-term success:

- **Depict Success:** Consider the advantages and favorable improvements you'll encounter if you accomplish your objectives. Visualizing accomplishment may inspire you in a significant way.

- **Support System** Tell your family and friends about your wellness goal so they can support you and help you stay on track.

- **Rewards:** Take into account establishing a system of rewards for achieving milestones. When you accomplish a task, reward yourself with something nice.

- **Consistency:** Integrate your health regimen into your daily life regularly. As habits are formed via consistency, it becomes simpler to remain motivated over time.

- Self-Awareness and Mindfulness Review your progress and the effects of your wellness plan regularly. Your dedication to the trip may be strengthened by this self-awareness.

The process of creating a natural health plan is dynamic and powerful. It gives you the ability to govern your health and general well-being as a woman. You can confidently manage your wellness path and attain the vibrant, holistic well-being you deserve by developing a tailored plan, establishing relevant objectives, monitoring your progress, and remaining inspired and responsible.

Chapter 11

Conclusion

I'm happy to hear that you finished "Natural Wellness Strategies for Women." We've set out on an exploration of natural and holistic methods of well-being throughout this ebook, customized especially to the special requirements and experiences of women. We'll summarize the most important lessons learned in this last chapter, motivate you to begin your natural health journey, and conclude by offering you some parting advice and a call to action.

1. A recap of the main points:

Keep in mind these crucial lessons as you consider the information and perceptions you learned from this ebook:

Physical, mental, emotional, and spiritual well-being are all included in the holistic concept of natural well-being.

- Make self-care a top priority, focusing on healthy eating, regular exercise, stress reduction, and enough sleep as the cornerstone of your wellness path.

- Recognize the significance of hormonal balance and menstrual health at various phases of life.

- Adopt a positive outlook and concentrate on energy and general well-being as you age.

- Investigate the world of dietary supplements and natural cures while constantly seeking medical advice.

- Make a tailored wellness plan, specify your objectives, monitor your progress, and maintain accountability.

2. Motivating Words of Advice for Readers Starting Their Natural Wellness Journey:

Your quest for well-being is a unique and powerful experience. ***Here are some words of inspiration to motivate you to take the first step:***

- By embracing your special female talents and attributes, you can organically alter your health and well-being.

- Keep in mind that even the smallest adjustments you make affect your general well-being.

  - Accept self-compassion and patience; remember that progress, not perfection, is what you are striving for.

  - Look for community and support, whether it comes from close friends, relatives, or those who share your outlook on life.

3. Final Reflections and Call to Action:

Consider these closing ideas as you read this ebook:

  It's never too late to begin or improve your natural health habits since improving your well-being is a lifetime endeavor.

  - Appreciate the uniqueness of who you are as a woman and embrace the beauty of your personality.

  - Act right now. Whether you're just starting on your health journey or perfecting your current routines, each step you take will help you get closer to a life that is vibrant and in balance.

We would like to conclude by inviting you to enthusiastically begin your natural health journey and to make a strong commitment to promoting your physical, mental, and emotional well-being. You may grow and thrive and live a life that emanates natural well-being, vigor, and overall harmony by implementing the ideas and methods covered in this booklet into your routine. Your adventure begins right now, so welcome it with an empowered heart and open arms.